Health Matters
Exercise and Your Health

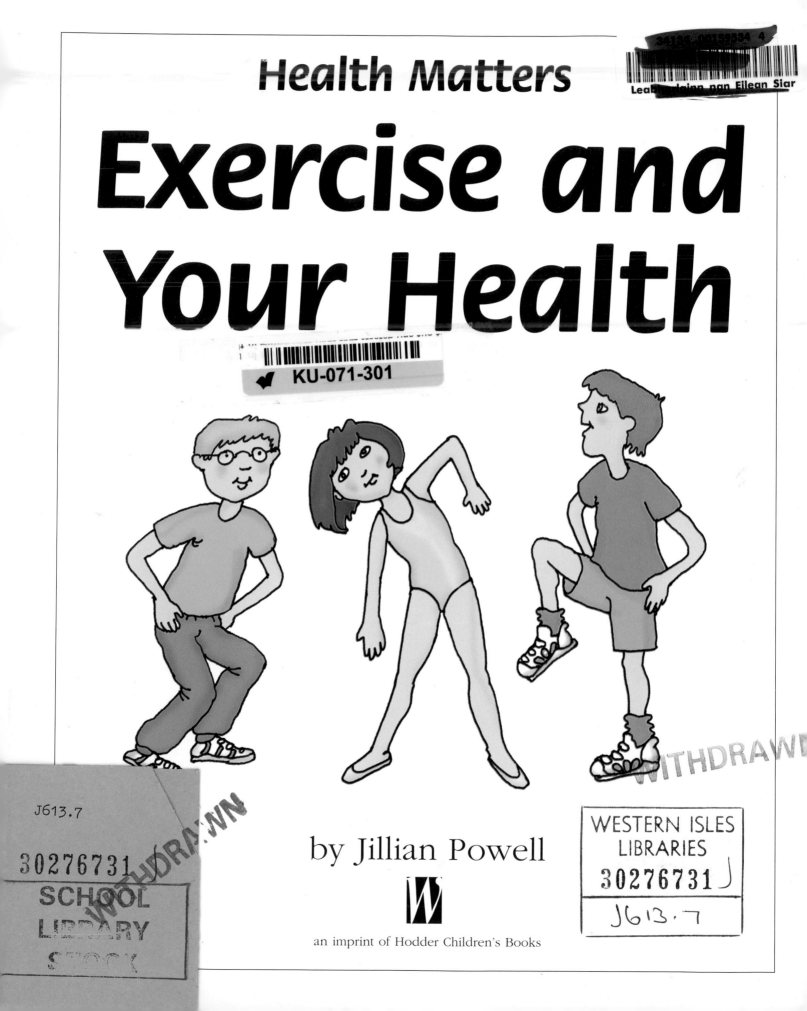

by Jillian Powell

an imprint of Hodder Children's Books

Titles in the series

Drugs and Your Health
Exercise and Your Health
Food and Your Health
Hygiene and Your Health

Editor: Sarah Doughty
Book editor: Penny McDowell
Design: Sterling Associates
Illustrations: Jan Sterling
Cover design: Tony Fleetwood
Cover photo: Stone (Joe McBride)

First published in Great Britain in 1997 by
Wayland Publishers Ltd

This paperback edition published in 2002 by
Hodder Wayland, an imprint of Hodder Children's Books

Hodder Children's Books
A division of Hodder Headline Limited
338 Euston Road, London NW1 3BH

British Library Cataloguing in Publication Data
Powell, Jillian
Exercise and Your Health – (Health matters)
1. Exercise – Juvenile literature
I. Title
613.7

ISBN 0 7502 4179 9

Printed in Hong Kong

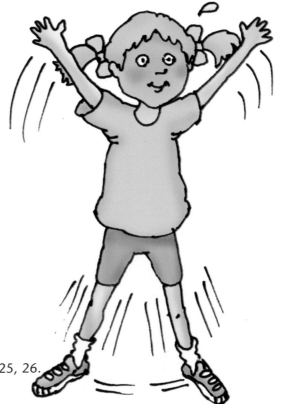

Picture acknowledgements
Action Plus 18, 28, 29; Tony Stone 7, 23; Wayland Picture
Library/(Chris Fairclough) 4, 6, 11, 14 (top), 17, 19, 22, 24, 25, 26.
All other photographs Wayland Picture Library.

Contents

Exercise is good for you

Your body is like an amazing machine. It needs to be used to keep it working well.

Exercise keeps your body strong and fit. Fitness means having the energy to work and play and do all the things you want to do easily. Your body cannot store fitness. You need to exercise regularly to stay fit.

Using your muscles makes them stronger.

Your heart and lungs are muscles. They need exercise to keep them working well and to help you fight off illness and disease.

While you are still growing, exercise helps your body to make strong bones.

Exercise makes you feel and look better. It keeps your body a healthy weight by using energy from the food you eat.

When you exercise, your body makes chemicals called endorphins. They go to your brain and make you feel good.

Exercise helps you relax and sleep better. It is like a magic tonic for your body, but you need to take it every day.

You get fit by making healthy choices about what you do and what you eat.

Strength, stamina and suppleness

You need to do different kinds of exercise to be really fit. Exercises for strength make your muscles stronger so you can work different parts of your body without feeling weak.

Exercises for stamina make your heart and lungs stronger and help your blood flow easily round your body. Stamina is the ability to exercise for longer without getting tired or out of breath.

Exercises for suppleness help your muscles and joints move freely so you can bend and stretch and twist and turn without feeling stiff or sore.

Doing many different types of exercise will help every part of your body to work better.

How fast is a fit human?

A snail moves at 0.05 km per hour.

A human sprinter can run at 43.37 km per hour.

A racehorse can gallop at 69 km per hour.

A cheetah can run at 100 km per hour.

If you get out of breath running upstairs, you need to improve your stamina.

If it is hard to touch your toes, you need to improve your suppleness.

If your legs start to ache when you are cycling, you need to improve your strength.

Swimming can help people of all ages stay fit. The water helps to support your body so you do not hurt yourself. Swimming is good for people who are overweight and people who have disabilities.

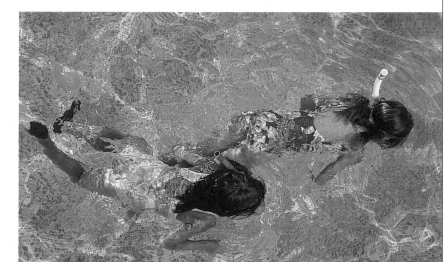

Food for energy

Food and drink give you energy. When you exercise, you use up lots of energy. Each day, you need to eat enough to provide about the same amount of energy that you use up.

If you eat too much and do not exercise enough, your body will store the extra energy as fat. If your body stores too much fat, you will be overweight and will be more likely to have health problems. If you do not eat enough, you will lose weight and you will not have enough energy.

Your body needs energy to grow and to work properly even when you are resting. When you are still growing, you need extra energy.

You can find out how much energy is stored in foods by looking at their labels. Energy is measured in kilocalories (kCal) or kiloJoules (kJ). Labels usually show how many kJ there are in 100 g of the food. Find out how much energy there is in some of your favourite foods.

A carrot contains 85 kJ of energy.

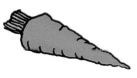

An apple contains 170 kJ of energy.

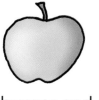

A burger and chips contains 3,000 kJ of energy.

A bowl of breakfast cereal and milk contains 700 kJ of energy.

An egg contains 380 kJ of energy.

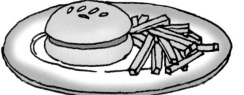

To use up the energy in a burger, large fries and a milk shake, you would need to run for three hours.

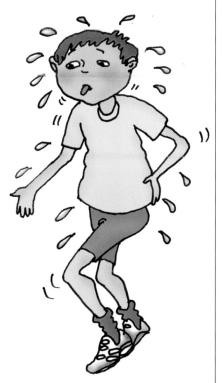

Foods that provide most energy are starchy carbohydrates, which should be the main part of each meal. Your body breaks down carbohydrates into glucose, which it can turn into energy.

Starchy carbohydrates include bread, pasta, potatoes, rice and cereals.

Warming up and cooling down

It is important to warm up and cool down every time you exercise. A warm-up gets your body ready for exercise. It helps your blood carry oxygen to your muscles so they are ready to work harder. You can warm up by marching or jogging on the spot and doing stretching exercises. Warm up for about five to ten minutes until you feel warm and you are breathing a bit faster than normal.

To cool down after exercising, do some slower movements until you are breathing normally again. Cooling down helps stop your muscles getting stiff and sore.

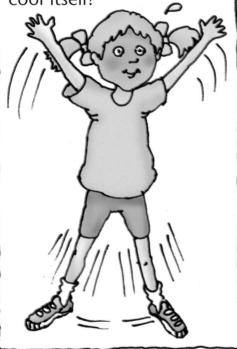

If you go red when you exercise, it is because blood is rushing to blood vessels near the surface of your skin so the skin can cool itself!

Stretching after exercise can help you to become more supple. Hold each stretch and count to ten.

It is important to warm up your muscles before exercising. If you exercise with cold muscles, you might hurt yourself. When muscles are warm, they are more stretchy and tear less easily.

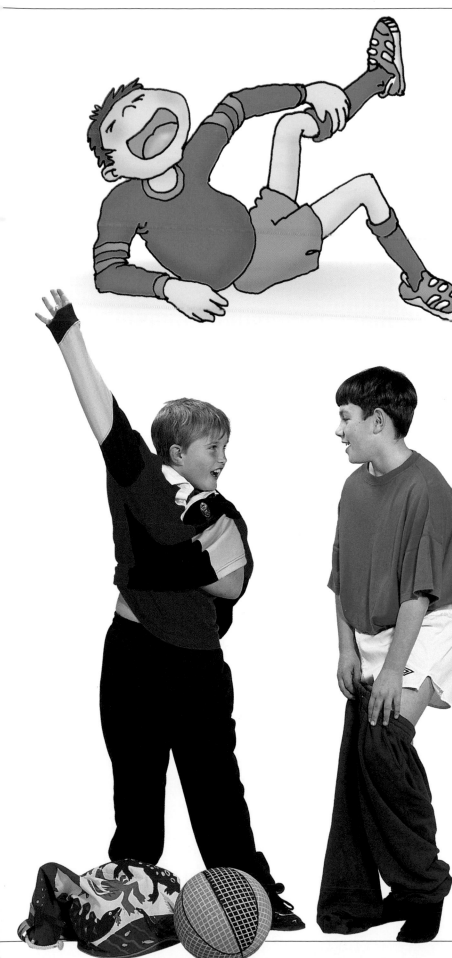

Leave a piece of Blu-Tack in the refrigerator until it is cold. Try tearing it. Now warm the Blu-Tack in your hands. Is it more stretchy when it is warm or cold? When does it tear easily?

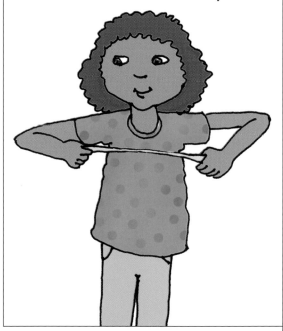

When you cool down, put on warm clothes as your body will be trying to get rid of the heat it made when you worked your muscles.

Bones and joints

Your skeleton is your body's framework. It is made up of lots of different bones. Bones give your body its shape and let you stand up and move about. They are strong and tough and protect the soft parts of your body.

Joints are places where your bones join together, like your knees and elbows. Joints help your body to move. Joints are held together by strong straps called ligaments. Shiny cartilage and a special fluid stop the bones from rubbing together and wearing out.

Your body is making new bone all the time. Children replace their skeletons about every two years.

Calcium, which we get from milk, dairy foods and some fruit and vegetables, helps to build strong bones.

The bones in your head protect your brain.

Some joints, like your shoulders, can move in lots of directions.

Your rib bones protect your heart and lungs.

Your largest bones are your thigh bones.

Human bone is very strong. A piece of bone 3 cm^2 can support 9 tonnes of weight.

You have about 206 bones in your body and about 100 moving joints.

Your smallest bones are in your ears. They are only the size of a match head.

The collarbone is the bone that people most often break.

Joints like your knees, can only bend in one direction.

Exercises for suppleness

Stretching exercises help keep your joints supple and stop them getting stiff. Being supple means you can do lots of different movements easily. You can bend, stretch and twist.

When you exercise, the muscles that work your joints are stretched so the joints can bend further. If you do not exercise, your muscles gradually get shorter and the joints become stiff. This makes you more likely to hurt yourself when you do sports.

Being supple helps you to do sports like volleyball, skateboarding, gymnastics and judo.

Gymnasts and dancers need to be very supple.

Stretching exercises are good for warming up and cooling down. Try:

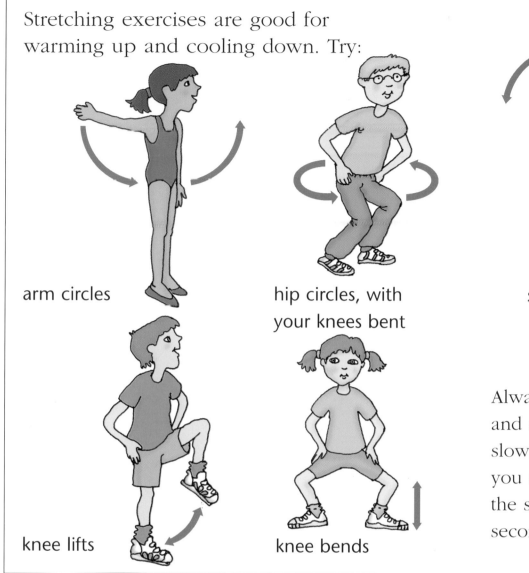

arm circles

hip circles, with your knees bent

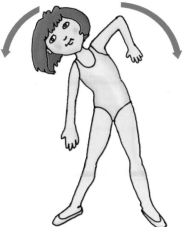

side stretches

knee lifts

knee bends

Always stretch gently and slowly. Breathe slowly and deeply as you stretch and hold the stretch for a few seconds.

To do a whole-body stretch, lie flat on your back with your legs slightly apart and your arms above your head. Stretch in both directions and count to ten.

When you try touching your toes, you may feel muscles pulling at the backs of your knees. Practise every day, stretching gently, and you will soon find you can bend further.

Muscles and how they work

When you exercise, you use your muscles to move your bones. To do this, muscles need energy from food and also oxygen from the air. You breathe in air and oxygen goes into your lungs then through your blood to your muscles.

Your biggest muscles are in your thighs and your smallest muscles are in your ears.

When you exercise, your muscles work harder so they need more oxygen. This is why you need to breathe faster when you are active.

You need about 200 muscles to walk, 30 muscles to raise an eyebrow and 15 muscles to smile.

Using your muscles helps make them stronger.

Some muscles go on working when you are asleep. Your heart pumps blood round your body and your lungs help you breathe.

There are over 600 muscles in your body.

Right: Pairs of muscles pull in opposite directions so you can bend or move different parts of your body.

One muscle shortens and pulls your arm one way. Its partner shortens to pull the arm back the other way.

If all the muscles in your body could pull together, they could move five elephants.

We all have muscles for waggling our ears but most of us never learn to use them.

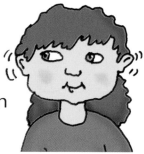

Below: If you have been ill and in hospital, you may need to do special exercises to strengthen your muscles. This is because your muscles become weak when they are not used.

Exercises for strength

You need to work your muscles to keep them strong. Strong muscles support your joints and help you to stand properly. They make it less likely that you will hurt yourself doing sports.

Strong arms help you to push, pull and lift. Strong legs mean you can run, climb and cycle. Different exercises help different muscles. Swimming is good for all your muscles. Running helps make your leg, back and shoulder muscles stronger.

Sports like discus throwing build up strength in the back, arms and shoulders.

Push-ups make the upper body stronger. Lie on your front with your hands under your shoulders and your toes pointing to the floor. Push with your arms to lift your body up, keeping your head down and your back straight.

Leg lifts make your back and hips stronger. Lie on your front and lift one leg then slowly lower it. Repeat with the other leg.

Start by doing these exercises five or six times, until you are strong enough to do more of them easily.

You can even exercise your fingers! Hold a soft rubber ball about 5 cm in diameter in the palm of your hand. Squeeze your fingers round the ball as hard as you can two or three times. Do the same with the other hand.

The heart and lungs

When you exercise, your heart beats faster and you take faster, deeper breaths. As you breathe in, air goes through your nose and mouth, down a tube into your lungs. Your lungs are like two sacks. They get bigger as they fill with air when you breathe in and smaller when you breathe out.

Oxygen from your lungs goes into your blood and is carried to your muscles. When you exercise, your lungs have to work harder to provide extra oxygen for your muscles.

Blood is pumped round your body by your heart. When you exercise, your heart pumps up to six times more blood than when you are resting.

Exercise makes your heart and lungs stronger.

You take in about 20,000 breaths every day.

Your lungs can hold enough air to fill about 18 drinks cans. Breathing deeply doubles the amount of air your lungs hold.

Heart

Heart facts

- Your heart beats about 100,000 times a day. It pumps about 43,000 litres of blood, enough to fill over 150 baths.
- Your blood vessels would reach twice round the Earth if you stretched them end to end.
- Your heart beats faster when you are nervous, for example, before an exam or a race.
- An adult's heart beats about 70–80 times each minute. A canary's heart beats 1,000 times a minute. An elephant's heart beats just 25 times a minute.

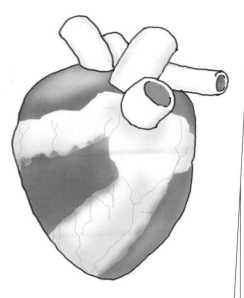

You can measure your pulse rate by finding your radial artery. It is under the skin on your wrist, just below your thumb. Place two fingertips over the artery and steady your hand with your thumb under your wrist. Use a stop watch to count the number of beats in 60 seconds. This will give you your resting pulse rate.

Check your pulse rate again, after you have done some exercise. What is the difference?

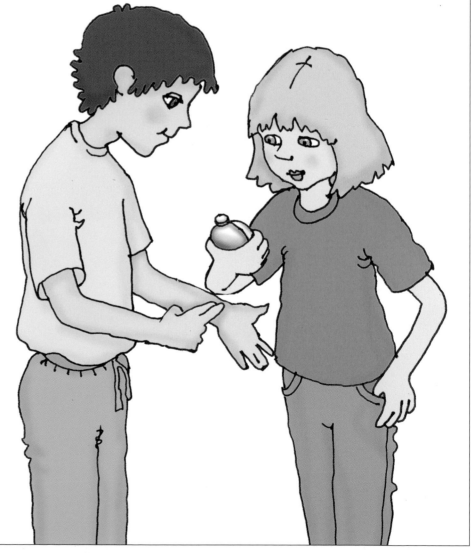

Aerobic exercise

Aerobic exercise makes your heart and lungs stronger. When you do aerobic exercise, you have to breathe in lots more air so your muscles get enough energy and oxygen to be able to work hard. When you are doing aerobic exercise, you should be breathing faster than usual but not so fast that you cannot talk.

Aerobic exercise helps to build stamina. As your stamina improves, you will be able to exercise for longer without getting too tired or out of breath.

Rollerblading, as well as running, swimming, cycling, dancing and skipping, all give you aerobic exercise.

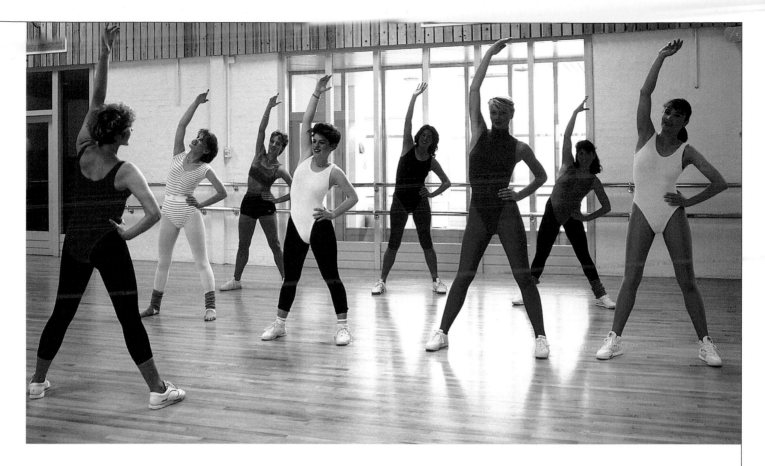

To stay fit, you need to do 20–30 minutes of aerobic exercise three times a week, including five minutes to warm up and five minutes to cool down.

Aerobics classes include jumping, jogging and stretching exercises.

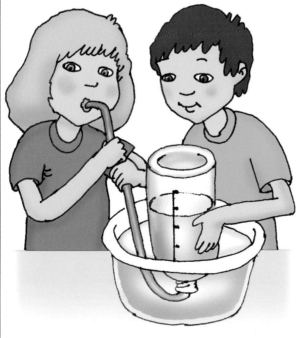

To test your breathing, mark a 2-litre plastic bottle in sections of 100 ml. Fill the bottle with water and cover the top with your hand. Then, turn the bottle upside-down in a bowl half-full of water. Get someone to hold the bottle while you feed a plastic tube into the neck, then try blowing through the other end of the tube as hard as you can.

How much water can you push out of the bottle with one big breath? The air in the bottle shows how much air you had in your lungs.

Exercise rules

It is important to keep your body safe and comfortable when you are exercising. Do not exercise just after a meal. Your stomach needs blood to help digest your food, so your muscles may not get enough blood to help them work properly. Do not exercise if you are feeling unwell or if you have a virus like a cold. Never exercise so hard that your muscles hurt or you feel dizzy, sick or tired.

If you are getting over an operation or illness or if you have asthma or diabetes, it is best to check with your doctor before exercising or doing sports.

Always drink plenty of water before and during exercise, especially in hot weather. This is to replace water you lose when you sweat.

Wearing the right clothes for exercise helps keep you safe.

Tracksuits are good for warming up and cooling down.

Cotton helps to keep you cool.

Sports fabrics like lycra are stretchy and comfortable.

Wear socks to stop your trainers rubbing your feet.

Trainers protect your feet and stop them getting sore. They must fit properly and have cushioned soles.

Wear layers so that you can take off clothes as your body gets warm. Put on warmer layers after cooling down.

As well as helmets, knee pads, elbow pads and wrist bands are important for sports like skateboarding and rollerblading.

Exercise plan

Exercise should be part of your daily life. Being active means walking or cycling sometimes rather than going everywhere by car or bus. Climb the stairs instead of taking the lift.

If you want to stay fit, avoid things that can harm your body, like smoking, taking drugs and eating too many fatty foods like chips, cakes and biscuits. Make sure that you eat plenty of fruit and vegetables.

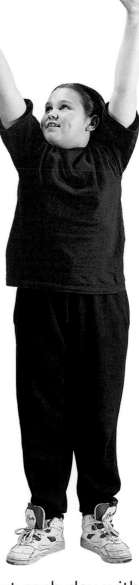

Start each day with a few minutes of stretching.

As well as doing things like watching television and using computers, make sure you get some exercise in the fresh air every day.

Rest is important for keeping fit. Sleep is your body's way of getting rest and repairing itself. Children need more sleep than adults.

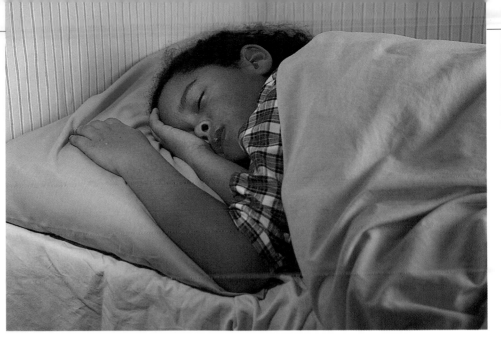

Draw up your own fitness programme.

Choose activities you enjoy and make a chart to show when you will do them each week. Leave boxes to tick when you complete each activity.

Try to include:

3 days a week:
5 minutes warm up
20 minutes aerobic exercise
5 minutes cool down

2 days a week:
15 minutes stretching exercises
15 minutes strength exercises
5 minutes cool down

1 day a week:
30 minutes of games or sports.

Don't forget to do some stretching every day!

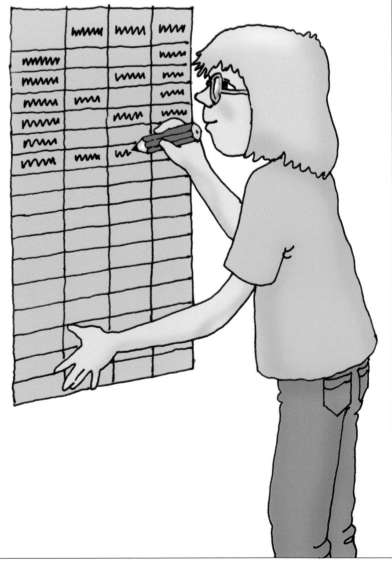

Exercise is fun!

It can be fun exercising with others. Check out the activities at your local sports and leisure centre or ask for information at the library. There are classes in activities like aerobics, swimming, judo, karate and gymnastics and team sports like soccer and volleyball. It is important to choose activities that you enjoy. Most sports centres have courts or pitches and equipment you can hire.

Joining in with team games like soccer, volleyball and basketball is a good way of making friends.

Try to get your family or friends to exercise with you. It is more fun if you exercise together.

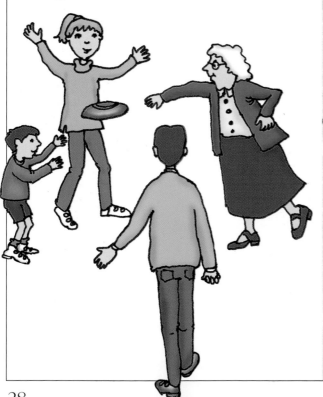

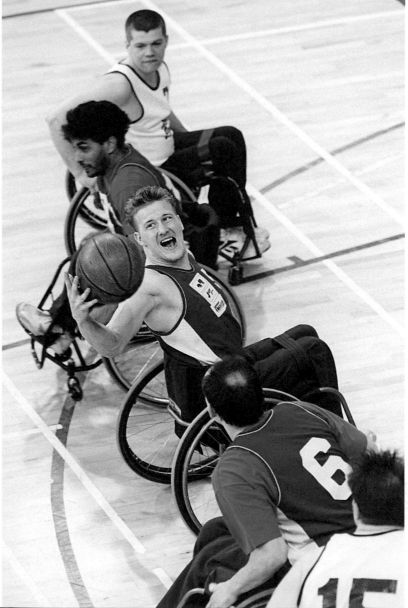

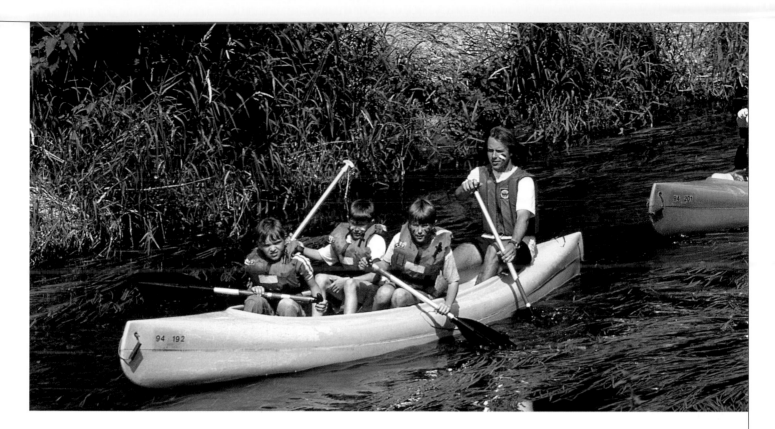

There are lots of sports clubs like cycling groups that organize day trips and holidays. You can choose from activity holidays including walking, swimming, tennis and cycling. You can learn new skills, like canoeing, windsurfing and climbing.

Walking is good exercise, as well as being fun, and it costs nothing!

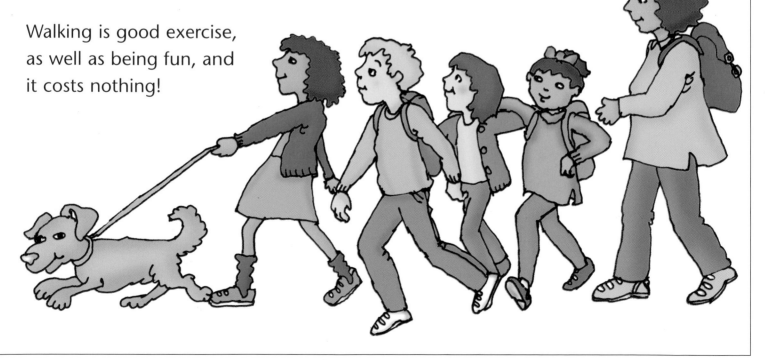

Glossary

Aerobic A type of exercise that uses lots of oxygen from the air and makes the heart and lungs stronger.

Artery A blood vessel carrying blood away from the heart.

Asthma Problems with breathing.

Blood vessels Tubes that carry blood round your body.

Carbohydrates Starchy or sugary foods that give you energy.

Diabetes A disease which means the body cannot control the amount of sugar glucose in the blood.

Digest The way in which the body breaks down food and uses it.

Kilocalories Measurements of the energy in food.

KiloJoules Measurements of the energy in food.

Stamina The ability to keep exercising without getting too tired or out of breath.

Suppleness Being able to move freely and easily.

Virus A type of disease.

Books to read

Body Maintenance Nicola Baxter (Health Education Authority, 1993)

Staying Healthy: Keep Fit! Miriam Moss (Wayland, 1992)

Running A Race Steve Parker (Franklin Watts, 1991)

Stay Fit Anne Qualter and John Quinn (Wayland, 1993)

For information about exercise

The Health Education Authority,
Hamilton House,
Mabledon Place,
London WC1H 9TX

British Heart Foundation,
14 Fitzhardinge Street,
London W1H 4DH

Index